Wired for Motion

Actions to Facilitate Your Unrestricted Movement and Fulfilling Life

Precious Hendrix

Copyright © by Precious Hendrix 2024. All rights reserved.

Wired for Motion

Table Of Contents

Introduction

I present you this book, full of tips on how to get your body ready for whatever that life throws at it, whether it is injury, age, or simply the everyday aches and pains that come with being a couch potato, gadget junkie, and coffee addict. You'll stop "throwing" your back out when you make the bed if you use this book as a guide. After a long day at work, you won't experience uncomfortable hunching over as you get out of a chair. Your shoulders will become more relaxed. You'll drop pounds and become less vulnerable to ailments like diabetes that are linked to it. Your vitality will return, your spine will become more stable, and your mind will clear. You'll be stronger, quicker, and less likely to injure your hamstrings or shoulders if you're an avid exerciser or athlete. Knee pain will subside. You'll be creating a very strong physique for yourself. You'll be doing it in a few rather surprising ways as well. People often get compartmentalized in their health (as well as in life) based on a variety of factors, including age, activity level, ability, and personal aches and pains. Regardless of our extracurricular pursuits, people are always battling against many factors such as gravity, technology addiction, food confusion, stress, sleep disturbance, and the unavoidable aging process. This book helps you become ready for the long haul. You'll read about some of the insights we've gained from high-achieving people across these pages. Even while such pearls of knowledge might be fascinating and useful, we're more interested in learning from individuals who have endured the longest. Not what distinguishes a great quarterback from a great quarterback, but rather what distinguishes the most resilient, everyday individuals.

Wired for Motion

Chapter 1

Raising Oneself From The Floor

When it comes to development, one of the most fundamental movements that youngsters engage in is getting up and down from the ground. We consider it a problem when we discover that children are unable to finish the work when they are of the age at which they should be ready to do so. Every so often, as we become older, we experience a change in behavior in which we begin to avoid being on the floor. Is that the case? Perhaps it is because there is a sofa that is more comfortable for you to sit on, perhaps it is just something that does not occur to you at all, or perhaps it is because you are afraid of not being able to get back up. Without regard to the reasons behind it, we are strong proponents of ensuring that everyone can get up from the floor at all times throughout their lives and that they never lose the ability to do so. Regardless of age, we have individuals working on this project now. The inability to get up off the ground should be seen as a problem, not as a reasonable side effect of age, and we should examine how we interact with children to fix this issue. We hope that by the time you finish reading this, you will have challenged yourself to go on the floor at least once a day. We are going to give you the top three reasons why we think this skill is so vital, and our goal is that you want to challenge yourself to do so.

The extent of one's motion

Wired for Motion

Raising Oneself from the Floor needs a substantial amount of range of motion in our joints to make that action feasible, a range of motion we don't generally test with everyday duties. Think about the things we do in our everyday lives: we sit in seats, we sit in our automobiles, we stroll about and we stand. If you examine the amount of range of motion required in our hips, knees, and ankles for those 4 tasks to happen, it's not very much. When it comes to our joints, we have the ability to achieve a far wider range of motion; yet, as the old saying goes, if you don't use it, you lose it. As a result, joints tend to become more rigid as we get older, and the range of motion that is accessible to us tends to decrease. But if getting up and down off the floor was deemed a daily exercise then we may be daily pushing back on joint stiffness and daily minimising the chance of tight joints and muscles as we age. This will consequently make us more mobile, more flexible, and more confident as we age.

Falling

Falling is a serious concern in the senior population, it may lead to fractured bones, and hospitalizations and snowball into a very large problem. Instead of teaching dread about falling and how things may go wrong, what if we focused more on how to age in a manner that makes you not as prone to falling? That way we may take an active role in our aging process and avoid living in dread all the time. Getting up off the floor may help you achieve precisely that. In a study of 307 senior individuals aged 75 and higher, not being able to get up from off the floor was a major predictor of severe fall-related injury. Practicing your ability to get up off the floor is a fantastic technique to not only lower your danger of falling but also provide you ideas on what to do if that does happen. We appreciate that most people reading this blog are under the age of 75 but we believe it is vital to know this knowledge now so it can allow you to know how to build yourself up for aging and do it in the best manner possible.

Mortality

Would the ground be an indicator of your mortality? Surprisingly, it is! Multiple research investigations have repeatedly shown this. In this research, 2002 persons aged 51 to 81 were examined on their capacity to get up from the ground on their own. After a 6-year follow-up, the persons with the least difficulty getting up from the ground had a reduced death rate. It seems to reason that this is the case, particularly given the increased range of motion and fall prevention benefits of standing up. So give it a try. Can you get up from the floor? If you can, wonderful! Keep it up. If you're struggling, figure out how you can make it happen. This might be done near a chair or coffee table so you can use your arms to lift yourself. Practice regularly, and as your range and strength improve, you will be pleasantly amazed at how easy this chore becomes! We want individuals to age smartly, so they know what they can do to best position themselves for the future. Never giving up the capacity to get up from the ground is a simple approach to remain active, strong, and live longer. Most of us don't even consider it while we're young. We just get down on the floor and stand up as required. Over time, a combination of back or joint problems and progressive muscle loss (sarcopenia) might make it difficult to get up from the floor without help. This becomes more difficult when we are alone and have nothing to cling to to climb back up. What is the greatest technique to get up from the floor? The most popular way employed by the elderly is to roll over onto their hands and knees, and then pull one leg forward beneath them. To return to standing, push off with your hands and legs. There's nothing wrong with utilizing this strategy, but I advocate alternating sides to ensure you're not simply strengthening one side of your body. Don't worry if it doesn't seem elegant; it just needs to be successful. Other ways to rise include staying on your backside and crossing your lower legs, or taking a broader stance; in any instance, you may use your hands for help if needed. If you can get up without using your hands, it is ideal, but it is not practicable. Other factors to consider are your general physical strength, balance, and agility. These are crucial components of your exercise program as you age, and they will help you with everyday tasks and when you need to get up from the floor. One of the challenges with aging is the steady loss of muscle mass, particularly in the legs. It will be useful to focus on workouts that strengthen the quadriceps, hip stabilizer muscles, glutes, lower leg muscles, and balance. Don't forget about the upper body; utilizing your chest, back, arms, shoulders, and core is equally vital. A full-body strength training plan that combines functional, mobility, and balancing exercises is very useful to anybody.

Some good workouts to start with are:
Wall sits, wall pushups. Rows with a band or hand weights. Plank (adjusted as required), Basic squats (adjusted as required) Balancing by standing on one foot Weighted or banded clamshells Bird dog (opposite arm and leg extensions while on hands and knees), and heel/calf lifts on a step or stairwell. For the best results, do these exercises two to three

times a week, with one to three sets of 10-15 repetitions each. This still allows you to fit in cardiovascular, stretching/flexibility, and mind/body workouts throughout the week. If you're unsure, ask a personal trainer who specializes in dealing with middle-aged and elderly people for assistance. Their role will be to assist you in learning the exercises, making adaptations, and working around any ailments to ensure you get the maximum benefit for your specific circumstance. Remember to keep active and strong as you become older. We cannot reverse the aging process, but we can surely slow it down.

Chapter 2

Breathe Easily

The respiratory center of the brain controls breathing, which is an autonomic function of the organism. When we are stressed, our breathing pattern and rate vary as part of the 'fight-or-flight reaction'. The stress reaction is another name for the "fight or flight" response phrase. It's what the body does when it prepares to face or escape danger. When used correctly, the stress reaction assists us in dealing with a variety of obstacles. However, difficulty arises when this reaction is continuously triggered by less significant, day-to-day occurrences such as financial difficulties, traffic congestion, work concerns, or relationship issues. Health issues are one of the consequences. A prominent example is excessive blood pressure, which is a significant risk factor for heart failure. Stress inhibits the immune system, making people more susceptible to colds and other infections. Furthermore, stress might cause anxiety and despair. We cannot and do not wish to avoid all causes of stress in our lives. However, we can build more effective responses to them. In the 1970s, Dr. Herbert Benson, a cardiologist at Harvard Medical School, was the first person to develop the relaxation response approach. Several approaches that elicit the relaxation response include a focus on breath. The first step is to practice deep breathing. Fortunately, we can consciously adjust our breathing. According to scientific research, managing your breath may aid in the management of stress and stress-related disorders. Breath control is also employed in techniques like yoga, tai chi, and meditation. Many individuals utilize breathing exercises to help them relax and decrease stress. Breathing's fundamental function is to absorb oxygen and exhale carbon dioxide via lung movement. The diaphragm (a strip of muscle underneath the lungs) and the muscles between the ribs are responsible for lung movement. When someone gets stressed, their breathing rhythm alters. A nervous individual often takes short, shallow breaths, moving air into and out of their lungs using their shoulders rather than their diaphragm. This breathing technique upsets the body's gas equilibrium. Shallow over-breathing, often known as hyperventilation, may prolong anxiety by exacerbating physical stress symptoms. Controlling your breathing might help alleviate some of these sensations. Breathing is possibly the most basic but complicated act we perform. It is a conscious thing if we want it to be, but the moment we stop thinking about it, it resumes on its own. One of our most pressing concerns is how things operate when they run on their own. Did we reset anything when we completed the breathing drill?

The benefit of deep breathing
In addition to being referred to as deep breathing, other names for it include abdominal breathing, belly breathing, diaphragmatic breathing, and timed respiration. Deep breathing causes your lungs to become full of air that is drawn in via your nose, and it also causes your lower abdomen to rise. A good many of us find deep breathing to be peculiar. There are various explanations for this. For one thing, the way people see their bodies has a negative impact on their ability to breathe in our culture. As a result of the perception that a flat stomach is attractive, both men and women do their best to tighten the muscles in their stomachs. This interferes with deep breathing

and eventually makes "shallow chest breathing" seem normal, causing tension and worry. The diaphragm's range of motion is restricted when shallow breathing is performed. When oxygen is not delivered to the lower area of the lungs, it is not properly distributed. Because of this, you can have feelings of shortness of breath and agitation. By promoting full oxygen exchange, or the beneficial trade of entering oxygen for leaving carbon dioxide, deep abdominal breathing works to promote complete oxygen exchange. Not unexpectedly, it has the potential to slow down the heart rate and either lower or maintain blood pressure.

Practising breath focus

Breath concentration allows you to concentrate on calm, deep breathing while disengaging from distracting ideas and sensations. It's particularly useful if you tend to hold your stomach.

First Steps: Find a quiet, comfortable spot to sit or lie down. First, take a regular breath. Then take a deep breath: Inhale gently through your nose, allowing your chest and lower abdomen to rise as you fill your lungs. Allow your abdomen to stretch entirely. Now, exhale gently via your mouth (or nose, if that seems more natural). After completing the preceding stages, practice regulated breathing daily. As you sit comfortably with your eyes closed, combine deep breathing with beneficial images and possibly a focal word or phrase to help you relax.

How to induce the relaxation response

1. Progressive muscular relaxation.

2. Mindfulness meditation.

3. Yoga, Tai Chi, and Qi Gong.

4. Repetitive Prayer

5. Guided Imagery

Establishing a schedule

To find the most effective relaxation method for you, you may want to experiment with a few various approaches. Additionally, you will have options if your preferred strategy doesn't work for you or if you just want something else. Also, you may find the following advice useful:

1. Select a particular spot where you may relax and be alone while sitting or lying down.

2. Go easy on the effort. That could simply make you tense.

3. Also, avoid becoming too submissive. Having a focal point is crucial for triggering the relaxation response, which is triggered by turning your attention from stressors to softer, slower rhythms.

4. To strengthen the feeling of ritual and create a habit, try practicing once or twice a day, always at the same time.

5. Aim to practice for ten to twenty minutes every day.

You breathe all day (and night), but how recently have you observed your intake and release of breath, particularly during physical activity? Now that you can't recall, let's get started. Why? Breathing exercises and modifying your breathing techniques according to the kind of exercise you're doing may have a good impact on your performance and overall well-being. According to Peloton teacher Nico Sarani, the act of just being aware of our breath, whether it be during yoga, other disciplines, or daily life, helps us tune into the present and the fleeting condition of our body and mind. Breath awareness offers us the ability to alter our mentality or state of well-being and to better understand who we are.

How Does Exercise Affect Breathing?
When you exercise, your heart and lungs are working hard: Your heart pumps oxygen to the muscles you need to power through that challenging Peloton class, while your lungs provide oxygen to your body and expel carbon dioxide. Your body begins to need more oxygen and produces more carbon dioxide when your muscles contract. The National Library of Medicine states that when you're at rest, you likely breathe in and out 15 times per minute, but while you're working out, your breathing will rise to 40 to 60 times per minute to handle the added demand. To provide your muscles with extra oxygen, your circulation will likewise quicken.

The Benefits of Correct Breathing During Exercise for Your Workouts
Your athletic performance may be significantly impacted by paying attention to your breathing while exercising. By breathing correctly, you're supplying oxygen to your muscles

as efficiently as possible, enabling you to work more in class and eventually achieve superior outcomes. However, you're more likely to take shallower, shorter breaths when you're not paying attention to your breathing, which results in less oxygen entering your lungs. Your blood pressure and pulse rate rise as a consequence, making it more difficult to engage in solid exercise and probably making you feel very uncomfortable.

Yoga Breathing Techniques

Yoga is an excellent place to start when improving breath awareness since it focuses more on the breath than most other hobbies do. However, it may still take some getting accustomed to altering your breathing patterns. Even while breathing is an essential part of yoga, don't worry too much about it in the beginning since the postures might take some time to get the hang of. You could eventually reach a point when movement and breath come together naturally, which has such a wonderful rhythm and sensation. Generally speaking, you should breathe in and out via your nose throughout a yoga session, making an effort to maintain the inhales and exhales equally lengthy and smooth. Breathing deeply and slowly may be beneficial both on and off the mat as it promotes mental and physical calmness. In yoga, this kind of breathing may also help you hold a posture longer or more comfortably, such as in Pigeon, which is an intensive pose.

Breathing During Cardiovascular Workout

When engaging in a cardiac exercise like jogging, it is recommended to breathe in through your nose and out through your mouth as evenly and continuously as you can. Similar to yogic breathing, it may take some time to become accustomed to this, particularly if you increase the intensity and find that you naturally want to breathe exclusively via your mouth. The run becomes simpler and easier with proper breathing. To assist the inhalation come more easily, concentrate more on completely exhaling through your mouth when you first start. If you can't feel your breathing, try saying "calm" and slow down. However, he thinks it's more crucial to have the nasal inhalation down pat if you're working out outside in the cold. He claims that the nose will warm the chilly oxygen, which is crucial since cold air may restrict or delay blood flow.

How to Breathe During Strength Training and Weightlifting

It's normal to question when, exactly, to exhale or inhale while lifting weights. When doing strength exercises, the exhale should occur with the concentric portion of the exercise (the resistance/effort) and the inhale should occur with the eccentric portion (the yielding component). To do a shoulder push, for example, you would exhale as you raised the dumbbells and inhale as you lowered them. Similarly, here's how to breathe while doing pushups: As you bring your body down to the floor, take a breath and exhale as you raise yourself back up. Similar to aerobic exercise, it is advised to breathe in through the nose and out through the mouth while doing strength training. For your muscles to remove waste products like lactate and CO2, they need oxygen in a strength class. During strength training, it's crucial to maintain proper breathing and oxygenation to avoid elevated blood pressure. To increase the amount of oxygen in your body, I would also advise breathing deeper into your stomach that is, all the way to your chest than you now are. Practicing mindful breathing is beneficial even when you're not working out. This information has shown to be a useful tool and can be seamlessly applied from the mat to everyday life. For this reason, I refer to yoga as a "lifestyle toolkit" at times. Whatever your illnesses or difficulties, yoga may help you get through them. When you wish to quiet your body and mind, she suggests that you should aim for longer and deeper exhales as a general rule of thumb. To get a more vigorous impact, do the opposite action and inhale deeply and for as long as you can.

Chapter 3

Stretch Your Hips

Opening up your hips is a basic hip extension. Every action that widens the angle between your thigh and the front of your pelvis causes you to extend your hips. If your hips are usually flexible, this movement can be manageable for you; nevertheless, without consistent training, it can become tight and especially challenging as you age. When you go from a sitting to a standing posture, your hips technically expand. Even though the muscles needed for these easy motions are among the biggest in the body, they nevertheless need to be regularly exercised to maintain their strength. Sitting too much, which tightens your hip flexor muscles and weakens your hamstrings, is a good way to see these strong muscles deteriorate. Neglecting these muscles might also occur from not consistently extending your hips fully. For instance, spinning doesn't need a complete hip extension, even though cycling is an excellent workout for muscular development. Naturally, you may keep your muscles flexible by stretching them regularly, but this is insufficient. Exercises that strengthen the body are essential. Hip extensions are utilized to help keep your pelvis stable during pedaling, climbing stairs, and walking. Hip extensions are easiest to practice as part of a morning routine. Simply lie on your side on a stable surface and lift one leg slowly, like a scissor. Yoga experts and the agile may do this by raising their legs to more extreme angles, but the best range of motion for this exercise is a shorter one, which puts the most strain on your targeted muscles.

Which Muscles Are Used in Hip Extensions?
The two muscles that are most important for hip extensions are your adductor magnus and gluteus medius. Since they work some of the strongest muscles, such as your powerful but often underutilized glutes and the extensors in your hips, hip extensions are very good for your strength and range of motion.

Hip extensions engage the deepest layer of your glutes. Primary muscles involved in hip extension include the long head, hamstrings, biceps femoris, semimembranosus, and semitendinosus.

Exercises for Hip Extension: Advantages for Glute Training

Alright, so well-known workouts like leg presses and squats will help you build, tone, and strengthen your glutes in addition to running and stepping machines. It may seem exaggerated to say that your glutes are neglected in your routine, but this is a big muscle group that needs more than just a basic squat to stay in shape. Though hip extensions are regarded as a standard exercise for glute training, they are undoubtedly helpful for increasing the strength and flexibility of the aforementioned extensors. The main muscle used in hip extensions is the gluteus maximus.

Exercises for Hip Extension That Work Best

Hip Extension Standing:

This is a single-joint workout that works your glutes, hamstrings, and lower back using only your hips. Starting from a standing stance, place one leg slightly in front of the other. Feel the strain in your hamstrings and butt as you push your rear leg out (backward) while leaning slightly forward and, if necessary, grabbing onto something for support. You may also do these by lifting your leg up and sideways in the same manner.

Extension of the Quadruple Hip

This engages your core a bit more while working roughly the same muscles as the standing hip extension. Starting on all fours, assume a table posture with your knees bent and at right angles to the floor, your back slightly arched. Raise one leg while maintaining a straight angle, elevating it as high as it will go in a gentle arching motion, then gently lowering it down to your starting position. Repeat with the other leg. The standing hip extension will be most felt in your lower back during this exercise.

Quadruple Pendulum Hip Extension

It is advisable to first become proficient in the simpler form of the quadruped hip extension before moving on to the more complex pendulum variation. You may build more strength and enhance your glutes and hamstrings by doing this exercise, which works best with more weight and resistance. Starting from a standing position, do a quadruped hip extension by using a leg curl machine or any other apparatus with a pendulum resistance lever. But this time, start with your leg up and contact the machine's lever while it's still at a straight angle. The idea here is to maintain the quadruped hip extension position and movements while pushing it out as you would in a leg press. Given the benefits of increasing weight, you can think about lowering the reps by doing more sets while raising the weight and resistance.

Swiss Ball Hip Extension

Wired for Motion

Swiss balls, often known as stability balls, are very useful. You may utilize one of them to strengthen your lower back, glutes, and hips. Start by placing a Swiss ball at your feet and reclining on your back on the floor. Place your heels and the back of your calf muscles on the Swiss ball while maintaining a firmly flat shoulder position on the mat. Since the main goal of this exercise is to increase stability, lift yourself by using your glutes and core to create the illusion of planking, with your heels on the ball and your shoulders on the ground. With a deliberate, gradual push, raise yourself to the planking posture. Then, bring yourself down to the ground by keeping your hips tight and your glutes engaged. Next, act again.

Machine for Hip Extension

Hip extension machines have a use, even though free weights are always preferable to machines for allowing a free and natural range of motion. All you have to do is use your strength; they take care of the movement and posture for you. Simple, huh? These devices need you to sit or stand and squeeze and expand your hips. The main benefit here is that it gives you the chance to raise the resistance and the weight you lift to produce bigger muscular growth and burn more calories overall. When it comes to producing the most speed and power possible during exercises like running and leaping, the posterior chain muscles—particularly the hip extensors—are crucial. Targeted hip extension activities often rank among a strength coach's top 5 exercises, and for this reason, squat, Olympic-style lift, deadlift, and lunge variants are regarded as foundation exercises in a strength and conditioning practitioner's program. The good morning, the 45° back extension, and the horizontal back extension are three focused hip extension exercises that are often done in sports weight rooms. The three exercises may all be classified as "hip dominant lifts" since their principal action is on the hip joint, provided that they are executed by flexing and extending the hips while keeping the spine and pelvis somewhat neutral. These exercises might be called "straight-leg hip extension exercises" since they do not involve a significant bending of the knees. It seems that the aforementioned hip extension exercises are interchangeable because of their comparable movement patterns. Stated differently, practitioners of strength and conditioning would generally presume that there is little variation in the execution and required training adaptations across the three exercises. However, there hasn't been a biomechanical investigation of these variants in the literature yet, so any conclusions about their interchangeability are, at most, theoretical. Strength coaches must create programs that translate to athletic performance at the highest level. Using the dynamic correspondence principle is one method to try to optimize training transfer. According to Siff, dynamic correspondence refers to the degree to which the methods of specialized strength training tailored to a particular sport align with the way the neuromuscular system functions in that particular activity. The emphasized area of force generation is one of the tenets of dynamic correspondence. One could argue that the different hip extension exercises are more suited to transfer more toward specific sports actions and result in unique structural adaptations if it were demonstrated that the good morning, 45° back extension, and horizontal back extension workouts resulted in various intensified areas of force generation according to the orientation of the human body in relation to space. Additionally, including these workouts into a training regimen may work in concert with sports requiring high power generation at various hip angles.

Exercises for hip extension are not all made equal. The human body's location on the ground affects the external torque. Exercises for standing hip extension that include a 90° bend forward show the maximum instantaneous torque. Exercises using hip extension at a 45° angle provide more constant amounts of immediate torque throughout the workout. When the hips are stretched, horizontal hip extension exercises provide the maximum degree of immediate torque. This little essay leads one to the reasonable conclusion that to maximize hip strength balance across the whole range of motion, a variety of hip extension exercises should be done. Additionally, it could be necessary to evaluate athletes across their whole range of motion to identify any strength deficiencies. This would allow for more accurate strength diagnosis and customized training plans. Lastly, a higher level of comprehension of training and exaggerated force/torque generation in connection to the activity or event of interest is required of the strength and conditioning practitioner. That is, exercise selection must be carefully considered for the best transfer from the strength and conditioning facility to the competitive environment (dynamic correspondence). To determine real-life hip extension moments, further research using force plates, electromyography, and 3D motion capture should be carried out. Further studies should be carried out to ascertain if the different hip extension workouts result in distinct structural changes that transfer to functional activities like running and leaping. Your whole range of motion is significantly influenced by your hips. Your capacity to walk and carry out activities of daily life may be impacted by hip issues brought on by chronic illnesses or accidents. Simple tasks might be difficult if you have a hip issue that affects your movement or creates discomfort. It may be difficult or impossible to walk, get out of bed, sit and stand for extended periods, or do household duties. The mobility of the hips may be impacted by many disorders. The good news is that there are hip-related surgical and nonsurgical therapies available to help lower discomfort and increase hip range of motion.

Anatomy of the hips
Among the biggest joints in the body is the hip. It is a "ball-and-socket" joint made up of the femur, a thighbone, and the acetabulum, a portion of the pelvis. To provide cushioning, cartilage covers the surface of the bones. The synovium, a lining, covers the surface of the joint. Hip mobility may be decreased if any of these hip components sustain damage as a result of an accident, misuse, or long-term illness.

Hip mobility-related conditions
The following circumstances may make it more difficult for you to move your hip:

1. Bursitis in the hips

2. Arthritis of the hip

3. Tendinitis in the hip

Bursitis in the hips

Hip mobility problems may result from hip bursitis, a painful inflammation of the bursae around the hip. Although direct damage or infection may also be the reason, repeated usage and overstressing the tissues around your hip joints are the most prevalent causes. In most cases, bursitis resolves on its own with rest and physical therapy. Surgery may be advised by medical professionals if your bursitis-related hip discomfort or immobility is severe or long-lasting.

Arthritis in the hips

Hip arthritis is an inflammatory condition that results in stiffness and discomfort in the hip joints. Hip mobility may be impacted by hip arthritis, making hip movement more challenging. It may be difficult to move your arms, sit comfortably, or do other everyday duties if you have severe hip arthritis. Physical therapy is a crucial first step for persons with arthritis, even if surgery or medication may be required for others. If you have hip arthritis, physical therapy may help you become more mobile in your hips.

Tendinitis in the hips

Hip tendonitis, also called hip flexor tendonitis, is the result of irritation or inflammation of the tendon that connects the iliopsoas muscles, which flex the hip. It also makes you uncomfortable and less mobile. Tendonitis is often brought on by frequent repetitive actions that overstress a tendon, such as playing sports like hockey, sprinting, or swimming, or engaging in high-impact exercises like spin classes. Painkillers, physical therapy, and rest are common treatments for hip tendonitis. In extreme circumstances, your physician could advise surgery.

Chapter 4

Consume Food As If It Will Last A Lifetime

It's normal for people to age throughout their lives. However, growing older does not equal developing typical aging-related conditions including osteoporosis, cardiovascular events, or neurological disorders. Our daily decisions about our food, exercise routines, and interpersonal relationships hold the secret to feeling younger, stronger, and healthier. Your life expectancy may be extended by eating a healthy diet and doing frequent exercise. Your chance of developing certain illnesses may also be increased by other variables, such as binge eating and excessive alcohol consumption. Eating is a vital component of self-care. Honestly, feeding your body nutrient-rich meals that promote optimal well-being is one of the BEST ways to love and appreciate oneself. We all need to eat, thus food serves as another common bond. Food is the universal language of celebration, social interaction, and self-nourishment. Eating shouldn't be difficult since food is a basic human need. or monotonous. perhaps too much. It ought to be uncomplicated, satisfying, and joyful. The majority of us, however, struggle with our connection to food and our bodies, and years of struggle may leave us feeling hopeless, damaged, and powerless. That being said, this is untrue. I think that we have an opportunity to start knowing ourselves on a much deeper level because of our eating and food difficulties. Eating well is one of the simplest ways to begin living eternally. Since lifestyle factors account for the majority of top killers, eating healthfully may lower your risk of dying young. Although a healthy diet won't prevent death forever given the state of medical technology today, remember that you are only attempting to postpone it until this technology catches up. Once it does, the danger of major causes of mortality will be eliminated, the aging process will be significantly slowed down, and finally reversed. Eating a healthy diet might raise the amount you spend each week on groceries, but it can also make you feel more alert and energized while you're waiting to die. Living eternally will always involve some suffering, or should we say investment instead? Nevertheless, this anguish is only temporary. That 50-year window is little in comparison to the additional centuries or millennia you may attain; those decades of vegetables and low-fat meals will soon be forgotten. And if we still require food in a millennium, you can be confident that our inbuilt nanobots will take care of all the negative consequences for you. You may eat everything you want, even doughnuts, whenever you want. Any lifestyle may be transformed with a good diet. Here is a list of superfoods along with cooking ideas and each food's health advantages. You can eat everything you want and live a long, healthy life by following this approach.

1. Greens with dark leaves

Superfoods such as spinach, kale, dandelion greens, and arugula are essential in the diet of seniors. Vitamin K, which aids in blood clotting and may lessen bone fragility, is abundant in dark leafy greens. For a simple way to get your recommended daily dose of Vitamin K, sauté or toss these greens into a spaghetti sauce or salad!

2. Tea Leaves

In addition to helping with digestion, green tea helps increase metabolism. Several glasses of green tea might help ease constipation symptoms. As an alternative, you or the elderly person you are looking for may find that drinking a cup or two of green tea helps reduce hunger. Vitamins and minerals abound in green tea. Enjoy it served with a squeeze of lemon or honey!

3. Raspberries

Antioxidants included in blueberries aid in the prevention of heart disease. In addition to being tasty on their own, they may be added to yogurt for dessert or eaten with oatmeal for an additional fiber boost for the morning.

Wired for Motion

4. Fish
Omega-3 fatty acids abound in salmon. Your blood fat percentage is lowered by the omega-3 acids, reducing your risk of heart disease. Add a drizzle of olive oil, season to taste, and bake at 425 degrees for your salmon. For a satisfying dinner that is healthy and tastes wonderful, serve with a full grain (such as brown rice) and a green vegetable.

5. Calcium-fortified Orange Juice
Strong bones and teeth are not just made of milk; orange juice and calcium also contribute to this. This may be consumed in the same way as milk, but without the additional hormones included in cow's milk, in one glass. Oranges give fiber and vitamin D, while calcium maintains healthy bones.

6. Whole cereals
The high fiber content of whole grains aids in digestion and protects the body from certain illnesses. Oatmeal, brown rice, quinoa, and wheat germ are a few of the healthiest whole grains.

7. Lentils
When it comes to antioxidant content, beans rank top. In terms of calcium, vitamins, fiber, and protein per serving, red beans are higher. Black beans, kidney beans, pinto beans, and little red beans are all great options for having a high antioxidant content.

8. Cloves

Wired for Motion

When taken regularly as a supplement, cinnamon lowers total cholesterol in a way similar to that of statin medications. Cinnamon's ability to lower blood sugar levels by up to thirty percent and aid in the body's effective usage of insulin is another wonderful benefit

9. Cherry tomatoes

Tomatoes contain lycopene, an extremely potent antioxidant. Tomatoes, raw or cooked, lower the incidence of both prostate and gastrointestinal cancer, according to studies.

10. Cranberry

Strong antioxidant that packs a punch. It reduces the accumulation of cholesterol plaque and bad cholesterol. It is very important in the fight against heart disease. The best method to get the advantages of this potent fruit is to drink pomegranate juice.

11. Sweet potatoes

Sweet potatoes are very versatile foods that may be eaten as an appetizer, side dish, or even dessert since they are high in antioxidants and typically simple to digest! You won't be sorry if you try topping a salad with warm, freshly cooked sweet potatoes!

12. Granny Smiths

Apples offer numerous additional health advantages in addition to their high antioxidant content, particularly in the skin. Apples are excellent for digestion and may help decrease cholesterol because of their high soluble fiber content. Vitamin C is also included in apples, which helps to strengthen the immune system.

Wired for Motion

13. Asparagus

Similar to its companion, the tomato asparagus has a high Lycopene content. Furthermore, asparagus has a high vitamin A content, which is beneficial to the immune system and eye health. Asparagus soluble fiber has the added benefit of lowering cholesterol. This dish has it all!

14. Broccoli

Broccoli is rich in antioxidants and fiber, but it's also a powerful source of vitamins A, C, B9, and K. This vegetable is good for the whole body, including your bones, tissues, and immune system.

15. Chocolate Dark

Not to mention, this delicious delicacy is very beneficial to your immune system and heart. It may even reduce blood pressure, which lowers the risk of heart attacks and strokes. Moderate afternoon or late sun exposure has also been associated with beneficial sleep outcomes. The most significant aspect affecting our health and well-being is the food we consume. However, many of us still experience confusion, unhappiness, shame, and anxiety around our eating habits despite, or maybe because of a decades-long discussion about nutrition. In light of the COVID-19 epidemic, everyone must understand the significant impact that healthy eating choices may have on maintaining our health. Not only is the proper operation of our digestive systems in jeopardy. It's the intricate network of processes that exist inside every one of our body's cells and is collectively known as our immune system. Therefore, eating a healthy diet helps us not only run our daily lives smoothly but also defend against infections and germs. We are significantly more adept at protecting our bodies from harm and, if we do become sick, recovering rapidly.

Chapter 5

Discover Your Balance

Achieving equilibrium in every aspect of your life is the path to success. Developing your body's equilibrium is part of this. Gaining better balance gives you more power and coordination, enabling you to move freely and steadily. Increasing your stability, agility, and flexibility makes carrying out your regular activities simpler. It enhances your athletic ability as well. Paying attention to your equilibrium might also aid in concentration and mental clarity. Exercises for balancing target your legs, lower back, and core. Exercises that strengthen your lower body might also help you become more balanced. Exercises involving balance might be difficult at times, but they will get easier with time and practice. As the workouts become simpler, progressively increase the amount of repetitions. If you need supervision or help, particularly in the beginning, feel free to ask for it. You may change the workouts to suit your requirements and to make them harder or easier. To make the second side simpler, start with your nondominant side. If you want to evenly distribute your body over both sides, you may perform your nondominant side twice. Try doing the exercises with one or both eyes closed once you feel comfortable with them. You may not give your balance much thought until it fails you, or you could be practicing yoga and trying very hard not to fall out of the eagle position. However, balance is much more than merely being able to balance in a yoga studio on one leg. Ultimately, regardless of your age or degree of fitness, it's essential for everything you do.

Why Maintaining Balance Is Vital to Our Health
In addition to enhancing general health and enjoyment of life, balance is essential for avoiding aches, pains, and accidents. Our underappreciated capacity for balance plays a major role in our ability to do daily activities including jogging, walking, and getting out of a chair. Research indicates that the degree to which you can execute these mobility abilities accurately or badly indicates the likelihood that you may encounter more severe incidents such as hip fractures, falls, and hospital stays in the future. Improved balance allows you to respond swiftly, regain momentum, and halt under control. Your capacity to execute rapid muscular contractions decreases with aging at a

pace twice as fast as your overall strength. Furthermore, that deterioration may quicken if you're not making an effort to strengthen your balance via exercise.

The Real Mechanism of Balance
Muscle mass is necessary for balance when we run, walk, leap, or stand. In terms of how well you perform in day-to-day activities and everyday life, balance mostly has to do with your capacity to contract your muscles swiftly to stabilize or generate a desired movement. Our muscles not only provide us with strength but also maintain the alignment of our bones and joints, enabling us to stand erect. However, balance also requires the interplay of three main sensory systems:

1. The first is what is visible to us.

2. The second is somatosensory, which consists of nerve receptors that give us the ability to touch and feel objects as well as proprioception, or the awareness of our own body in space.

3. The vestibular system, a small but intricate inner ear system that reacts to gravity, is the third.

All three systems provide input, but the visual system is the one that most of us use most often. Upon seeing our surroundings and near surroundings, our brains send out a sequence of signals that serve as an instant, comforting reality check: everything around you is in order, and you are too. But for the same reason, during balancing training, we will instruct someone to shut their eyes. The other two senses may become more robust if the visual is removed.

How to Get and Keep a Healthy Balance
Age-related declines in the visual, somatosensory, and vestibular systems occur, and we start to lose that crucial muscle mass as early as our 30s. According to Tanvi Bhatt, PhD, associate professor of physical therapy at the University of Illinois Chicago's College of Applied Health Sciences, the deterioration starts very gradually but peaks around age 65. This is when practicing balance comes in handy. Making the right neuromuscular connections, that is, connections between your brain and muscles, is similar to learning to play an instrument, according to Jonathan Cane, an exercise physiologist and the creator of City Coach Multisport, a New York City endurance training company. Then, to prevent those connections from breaking down, you need to practice. Although your balance may vary from day to day due to injuries, muscle pain, weariness, and sleep deprivation, Bonhotal emphasizes that the most important thing is to practice balance regularly at least every other day, if not daily. To begin, try standing on one leg while brushing your teeth or cleaning up fallen things with one leg raised behind you (as you become better, push yourself even more by raising the lifted leg). Standing on one leg with your eyes closed for as long as you can until you lose balance (time it!), and then switching sides, is a simple and effective way to improve balance if you're limited on time, space, or energy. As you practice, notice that your time becomes longer.

In general, Bonhotal states that if you do exercises like these, you're already receiving a fair dose of balance training:

1. Single-leg workouts, such as step-ups

2. Exercises using split stances, such as lunges

3. Exercises involving an uneven load, such as moving or holding a weight only on one side

4. Core workouts

On the days when you don't do any of these, you may just require five to ten minutes of organized balance training if any of these are a regular component of your workout regimen. However, if you want to include more focused balance training into your routine, here are some fantastic exercises that focus on developing stability and balance.

Exercises for Balance

Alignment of the spine
Experts agree that optimal spinal alignment is necessary for effective, injury-free mobility. Comana suggests that you place your heels on a wall to check the alignment of your spine. Your tailbone, shoulder blades, and back of the head should all strike the wall in a neutral alignment, meaning they shouldn't be inclined either upward or downward.

Try this if, like the majority of us, you don't touch the wall in all three places:

Wired for Motion

Reach for a rolled-up beach towel or a 36-inch foam roller. Lay it lengthwise on the floor with your head, spine, and tailbone resting on top. If your head is tipped back, lay a second towel or a hard cushion below it. With your arms at your sides, flex your knees. Allow gravity to draw your shoulder blades down on each side as you lie there for five minutes. Until all three points can be contacted, try doing this twice a day and doing the wall check once a week.

Fixed Lunges

Put your feet hip-width apart to begin. Make a lunge by leaning forward and keeping your heel off the ground. Maintaining a straight spine, bend both knees and drop your back knee toward the floor. Raise yourself back up to the beginning position and repeat with the front leg of the other person. Repeat 10 times on each side, switching up which leg is in front. As you go, you may add weights if you'd like. Split squats, also known as isometric lunges Place your left foot firmly on the floor in front of you and begin on the floor in a half-kneeling posture with your right knee and shin down. (Verify that the hips and knees are in line and that both are at a 90-degree angle.) Maintaining your right foot planted on the ground, raise your right knee slightly above the floor and maintain this posture, which will resemble the lower portion of a stationary lunge. Maintain a raised chest throughout the hold to ensure that the shoulders and hips line up. Without stopping, increase the holding time to 30 seconds by starting with five to ten seconds for each leg. Make two or three sets for each leg. To make it more difficult, gradually increase the amount until you can hold for five minutes on each leg.

Calf Raises / Heel Raises

Stand upright with your feet no wider than hip width apart. In case you need to grab onto anything for support, stand close to a wall, the back of a solid chair, a railing, or any other surface. Maintain a neutral spine by using your core and lifting both heels off the ground while maintaining control and rising into the balls of your feet. Avoid curving your back or forward. After pausing for a time at the top, slowly and deliberately descend your heels down to the floor (don't hurry this phase of the exercise; it demands balance). Do three sets of ten repetitions in total.

The tightrope walk, or heel-toe walk

Move like you're on a tightrope by maintaining control and walking in a straight line: Put your front foot's heel right in front of your rear foot's toe with no gap between them for every stride. After ten steps in one direction, reverse course and take ten steps back to your starting point. Repeat three times (one set is there and back). This may be made more difficult by looking forward rather than down at your feet, or by going backward.

Standing on one leg with closed eyes

Begin by standing squarely in a neutral posture next to a wall or other sturdy object that you may grab onto if necessary. Shut your eyes, then lift one foot off the ground just a little bit, you don't have to elevate it that high, and keep it there for as long as you can. Set a timer, mentally count, or count the cycles of your breaths. As you become better, work your way up to 20 or 30 seconds, starting with only 5 to 10 seconds.

Romanian Single-Leg Deadlift

Put your feet hip-width apart to begin. If you can, try striking balance on one foot. Start with one foot roughly two foot-lengths behind the other if you are unstable. The front leg, or supporting leg, should have its knee slightly bent. Hold your back straight and stretch both arms forward toward the floor, hanging from the hips. Once again, rinse and repeat with the other foot. If you'd like, increase the weight as you go.

Tall Plank Featuring Shoulder Taps

With your hands slightly wider than your shoulders, begin in the high plank posture on the floor. Bring your knees to the floor, much as you would for a modified push-up posture, to make it simpler. Lift your right hand off the ground, engage your core, and touch your left shoulder. Continue to alternately touch one hand to the opposing shoulder as you slowly release your hand to the ground. Make an effort not to allow your hips to sway or your weight to move. Perform ten repetitions on each side. Having trouble staying balanced? Spread your feet apart. Bring your feet together or do the exercise with one foot off the ground for added difficulty.

Canines Avian

positioned your knees and shoulders under your hips. Lift and stretch your left arm forward while simultaneously extending your right leg behind you by using your core. As you elevate each leg, maintain a straight, table-like back, don't twist it, doing this exercise in front of a mirror for added benefit. Hold for five times. Repeat with the other leg and arm. Perform five repetitions on each side, switching sides.

Curtsy Lunge With An Indirect Bite

Place your elbows out wide and connect your fingers to your ears while keeping your feet hip-width apart. This is a curtsy lunge. Cross your right leg behind you and drop the right knee till it is one to three inches off the ground. Maintaining your balance and weight on your left leg, raise your right leg to your right elbow while bending your body slightly to the right (into an oblique crunch when standing). Be cautious not to twist your hips. Start with a release, then repeat 12 times. Repeat on the other side.

Step-Ups with Just One Leg

Step onto an exercise box, step, or set of steps with your feet hip-width apart. Raise your left knee to around hip height with your right leg. For a little while, hold at the top without putting your left foot on the box. To return to the beginning position, step back down to the floor with your left foot first, then your right. After ten repetitions, swap legs and do ten more reps. Each performs three sets.

Crunching Up While Putting Your Legs Up

Place your feet together as you stand. With your knee bent at a 90-degree angle, raise your left leg to hip height in front of you while shifting your weight to the right foot. Raise your hands straight up over your head and firmly push them together. Clap your hands beneath your left leg while bending your body forward. Then, release the grip and lift your arms back up above, keeping your left knee elevated. On one side, repeat ten claps (without placing your left foot down). Repeat on the other side.

Tree Position

Take a neutral standing stance to begin. Taking a breath, press the inside of your left leg to the bottom of your right foot. Breathe out while extending your right knee wide to the side. While holding this stance for 20 seconds, take deep breaths. Lean your left foot on your right calf and repeat on the other side.

How Age Affects Balance

Age-related balance issues are often associated with pleasantly wobbly grandparents, but they may affect us even before we become Social Security eligible. Visual acuity, which includes peripheral vision and depth perception, starts to decline with age, and "the proprioceptors embedded throughout the body become less sensitive," according to Comana. As a result, you are not learning new knowledge as fast or precisely, and you respond to situations that may cause you to stumble more slowly. We may get nervous when we see ourselves as sluggish, which might be another reason why the young bounce in our stride becomes a cautious shuffle. Additionally, the inner ear's vestibular nerve endings tend to deteriorate with time. Regardless of our age, technology is upsetting our equilibrium, which only makes things more complicated. Put it down to the all-too-common practice of looking at our phones all the time. Someone may view 50 feet ahead of them instead of 300 feet due to a crooked neck. Furthermore, muscles and stability are weakened by the physical imbalance. However, these consequences are becoming more noticeable in younger people now that phones and computers are around. The good news is that you can maintain or improve your balance at any age with consistent practice.

Wired for Motion

Chapter 6

Sleep Is Your Superpower Unleash It

Sleep often suffers in today's fast-paced society due to hectic activities. But what if you could develop a superpower that enhances every element of your life just by making getting enough sleep a priority? Many of us have thought of "pulling an all-nighter" or staying up late to meet deadlines at work, school, or other institutions. I am aware that I have. Perhaps doing so seems like a good and effective approach to do the "urgent" work at hand in the short term, but what long-term effects are you causing to your body? Do we ever give the urgent more weight than the essential at times? Even though you've probably heard that getting enough sleep is important, have you thought about it to see if there's anything you might be doing differently? Most of us often wait until something begins to negatively impact our lives before changing our way of living. Perhaps we "wake up" when a friend, family, or co-worker suffers from sleep deprivation. That's simply the way each of us is wired.

As a species, humans are inquisitive, inventive, and creative. Sometimes this characteristic might make ordinarily straightforward body processes like eating, walking, or sleeping more difficult or problematic. Things that were formerly thought of as a regular way of life become outdated with every new generation of innovations and difficulties. Consider the following inquiries for yourself:

1. What is the duration of your sleep?

2. When do you usually go to sleep?

3. Do you experience deep, restorative sleep that is uninterrupted?

4. Do you ever check your phone when you wake up in the middle of the night? or see what time it is?

5. Do you use your phone to browse the internet or watch TV just before bed?

6. When you wake up, do you feel renewed, bright, and refreshed?

Many of your issues could have hints in your replies. The ease of these questions and the ease of their solutions will surprise a lot of us. Although the introduction of technology has undoubtedly improved our lives, too much of anything may be hazardous or even addicting. Everyone in the globe, both the younger generation and the elderly, is enamored with smartphones. In addition to smartphones, other things that have affected people's ability to sleep include televisions, employment, stress, financial concerns, and worry. People who gaze at blue light-emitting devices in the evening report difficulty waking up in the morning, a longer time to fall asleep, and less REM sleep, the stage of sleep during which dreams occur. Our body clock operates on a basic principle: when it's dark outside, your brain recognizes that it's nighttime, which is when you should go to bed. Your brain recognizes that it is time to get up when the morning light touches your eyelids. Hormones with intelligence can recognize these patterns. Melatonin, which is produced by the pineal gland, regulates sleep patterns in both seasonal and circadian cycles, which last twenty-four hours. The only time we get close to realizing the impact of these hormones, particularly melatonin, is when we suffer from jet lag, but otherwise, we don't pay much attention to them. Why is it that we should value sleep more? We typically remember knowledge better and perform better on memory-related activities when we get enough sleep. Our bodies need regular sleep times every day to repair and develop muscle, sanitize blood vessels and tissues, synthesize hormones, boost immunity, and keep our moods steady. Chronic sleep deprivation has been associated with a higher risk of high blood pressure, diabetes, cancer, stroke, heart disease, dementia, renal disease, mental health issues, obesity, and weight gain. It is concerning that people are not aware of the negative effects sleep deprivation has on both mental and physical health. Seventy-five percent of individuals with depression exhibit symptoms of insomnia, and many also have hypersomnia and excessive daytime drowsiness. Some of us take satisfaction in staying up late to get more work done, along

Wired for Motion

with our friends, colleagues, and peers. Although few people are aware of or have firsthand experience with the negative effects of sleep deprivation on general productivity at work, it is seldom discussed about unethical behavior, decision-making, abrupt mood changes, and creative thinking. Every working day may provide several obstacles for people with irregular sleep patterns, which those who get a full night's sleep might not be aware of. An adult needs between seven and nine hours of sleep every night to function well. This sleep may make you more focused, alert, empathetic, and creative, and have a happier, more optimistic outlook on life. Food is important since people can go far longer without it than they can without sleep. Have you ever wondered why going to bed is often a quick fix for a variety of issues? Sleep is one of the most underappreciated remedies and the body's true overnight healer. It can solve a lot of issues. Since I can start and finish work early, eat supper before 7 o'clock, which I couldn't do for years, and go to bed before 9:30 pm. I have personally seen a significant improvement in my health and general well-being. My ability to strike a healthy work-life balance has improved my ability to sleep well, keep a healthy lifestyle, and concentrate better at work. In the past, particularly when I was younger, I took sleep for granted. Now that I know what I do, I wholeheartedly agree with the adage that "being wealthy, wise, and healthy starts early in life.

Insufficient Sleep Is Your Death Contract

You won't believe how much difficulty a bad night's sleep can cause. Sleep is an essential component of good health since it is the foundation of your body's natural ability to heal and regenerate. Do you have high blood pressure, diabetes, obesity, cancer, coronary artery disease, stroke, depression, cognitive impairment, or Alzheimer's disease? You need to make a bigger investment in both the amount and quality of your sleep. You may save up to 40% of your resources if you get enough sleep. Numerous global surveys indicate that over one-third (33.8%) of the world's population has irregular sleep patterns. Since the world is becoming a more capitalist place, most individuals prioritize achieving financial success over maintaining healthy sleeping patterns. This describes the current global epidemiological change that is being witnessed. Non-communicable illnesses are becoming more prevalent in our culture. Examples include cancer, obesity, heart disease, genetic problems, and obesity. Compared to 25% of males, 40% of women will have sleep abnormalities. The most often disregarded essential component of wellness is sleep. Nearly no one is aware of how crucial the ability to get restful sleep is. It is foolish to strive for productivity while getting little sleep. It is also erroneous to believe that maintaining excellent health via food and exercise alone is possible. Finally, it is a catastrophe to want to stay youthful and energetic while getting insufficient sleep. Without getting enough good-quality sleep, we cannot expect to live longer because: "Restorative Sleep," or a full cycle of sleep, accounts for 80% of the body's healing process. I want you to think twice about the way you sleep.

1. Being sleepy slows down response times, making it harder to respond quickly in an emergency. In the USA, it is to blame for over 100,000 accidents annually and a startling 1,550 fatalities from crashes. A thousand mishaps in medicine and much more

2. Your creativity suffers when you sleep less. logic, focus, alertness, attention, and problem-solving skills. A healthy sleep pattern is crucial for helping the mind solidify memories. One bit of advice: make sure you get adequate sleep if you're studying a new idea.

3. The occurrence of the aforementioned illnesses is linked to decreased sleep.

4. Did you realize that getting too little sleep reduces libido? Men with sleep apnea have been shown to have low testosterone levels.

5. Depression and anxiety are most frequently linked to sleep durations of fewer than six hours every night. Resolving sleep issues can lessen the signs and symptoms of depression.

6. You want to appear gorgeous; sleep deprivation ages the skin. Cortisol, the stress hormone, is produced in greater amounts the less sleep there is. This hormone causes a significant reduction in skin suppleness by breaking down collagen in the skin. Additionally, during stages 3 and 4 of slow-wave sleep, the growth hormone, the primary hormone that supports cellular and organ repair is produced.

7. Sleep deprivation affects judgment and causes forgetfulness. Unaware of this, the majority of individuals believe they are making the proper choices. Being sleep-deprived causes emotional and illogical behavior. Getting enough sleep is crucial for mental health.

8. You're trying to get in shape. Good news: 7 to 8 hours of sleep is what you should aim for. Less than six hours of sleep causes the hormones Ghrelin, which promotes hunger, and Leptin, which mimics appetite, to be secreted in greater amounts.

Your most economical and straightforward tactic to seize the lead will be getting a good night's sleep while you concentrate on reaching your objectives. DO basic things to get exceptional outcomes. How can you create healthy sleeping habits from a young age?

Proven strategies to ensure a restful night's sleep.

1. Even on weekends, wake up at the same hour every day.
Your circadian rhythms will be aided by this, enabling you to naturally go to sleep and get up at the same time every day. Circadian rhythms: what are they? Your body clock uses these biological processes to determine when it is time for you to get up and go to sleep.

2. Refrain from using your phone after dark.
Our brains may be signaled by a bright light to remain alert, and the continual pinging that occurs when we are tagged in a new post or get a message from a buddy keeps our minds active. To avoid the blue light, it's a good idea to turn off or put your phone in night mode. You should also keep it away from you to lessen temptation.

3. Consume caffeine in the morning rather than in the afternoon.

Did you know that caffeine has a half-life of around five to six hours? That's how long it takes your body to break down and get rid of half of the caffeine. Therefore, by 9 pm the quantity of caffeine in your system will still be half what it was at 3 pm if you had a cup of coffee. The length of time varies based on your age, weight, and general health. Pregnant women may need up to fifteen hours.

4. Be mindful that daytime naps are included in your overall sleep duration.
Because they need to wake up from a deeper sleep, daytime naps might make you feel sleepy. Additionally, naps taken after 2 pm throughout the day should be avoided since they might complicate nighttime sleep. Keep them under 20 minutes and before 2 pm, if necessary.

5. Verify the temperature in your room.
To ensure that you get the greatest possible sleep, make sure the room temperature is just perfect. It will be much simpler to fall asleep if your room is chilly, as opposed to heated. Adjusting the thermostat above or below the appropriate level might cause agitation and compromise the quality of your sleep.

6. Remain physically and mentally engaged.
Both mental and physical exercise may improve the quality of your sleep. Frequent exercise alters brain chemistry to enhance thinking, memory, and sleep quality. The most physiologically restorative sleep period, deep sleep, is prolonged when there is physical activity.

7. Be mindful of melancholy and distress

Sleep issues may be brought on by stress, worry, or sadness, or they might exacerbate pre-existing conditions. Were you aware that difficulty falling asleep, or insomnia, is a typical symptom of depression? You must distinguish a disrupted sleep cycle from other conditions.

8. Steer clear of workouts and hot showers too soon before bed.

Exercise late at night affects your body temperature, heart rate, and sleep pattern. Adrenaline, norepinephrine, and cortisol are the chemicals that keep your body running throughout a demanding workout; although this keeps you awake, it won't help you go to sleep. The same applies to shower or bath settings that are overly warm.

9. Steer clear of sleeping drugs; they don't improve sleep over time.

In the short term, a sleeping pill could help you stop having trouble sleeping, but it's crucial to make sure you know all there is to know about them. In the long term, they don't aid with sleep and may have negative health impacts. When you can, stay away from sedatives.

10. If you gasp for breath while you sleep or snore, or if you feel very tired throughout the day, see your doctor.

When you have obstructive sleep apnea, your upper airway narrows and blocks your breathing, preventing you from getting enough oxygen until you wake up and resume breathing. The only symptoms of sleep apnea you could experience if you don't have a companion to witness your snoring are excessive daytime tiredness or morning headaches.

If you're worried about your sleeping patterns, see your physician. Make getting enough sleep a priority and use some of the above advice to ensure that you receive the best possible night's sleep since sleep is essential for your general health and wellness.

Conclusion

Finally, if you want to live a meaningful life, you need to appreciate the positive things that are already in your life. The practice of expressing thankfulness has been shown to have several positive effects, including the enhancement of relationships, physical and emotional health, sleeping patterns, mental endurance, vitality, and general happiness. Being appreciative is one of the simplest and most effective things you can do. When you find that you are unable to find the desire to finish a job (or even begin one), you should think about the various reasons why you are having difficulty. The next step is to devise a strategy that will assist you in getting into motion. Always keep in mind that not every method is effective for every single person or in every single circumstance. Perform some behavioral tests to evaluate which tactics best help you attain your objectives. Problems with motivation are something that everyone faces at some point in their lives. On the other hand, what is important is how you react when you find yourself lacking drive. Be gentle to yourself, try out different methods that might boost your motivation, and if you find that you want assistance, don't hesitate to ask for it. Sometimes, being terrified of failure might be an indication of a more severe mental health disorder. Negative thinking may lead to serious health issues, and in the most extreme circumstances, it can even result in death. While the strategies in this book have been demonstrated to have a good influence on your unhindered journey to a fulfilled existence, they are for advice only. Readers should consider the counsel of appropriately certified health specialists if they have any worries concerning linked health problems or if negative thoughts are creating severe or chronic suffering. Health experts should also be contacted before any big change in diet or amounts of activity. In a word, an effective strategy to begin living more genuinely is to envision the life you want and discover the components that energize you and make you happy. While happiness is not the goal, but a by-product of a life well lived, you may still make joyful experiences with enduring significance.